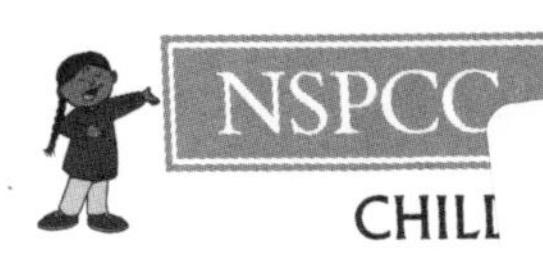

CHILL

First-tir ... ~ııT

by

Faye Corlett

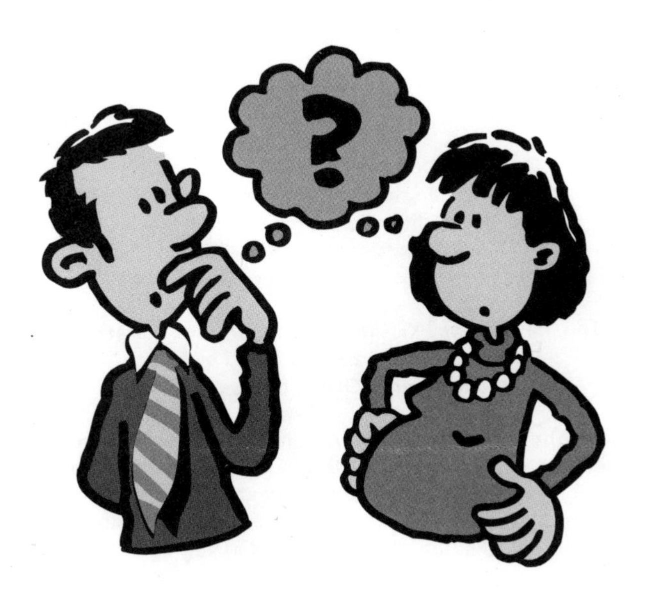

EGMONT WORLD LIMITED

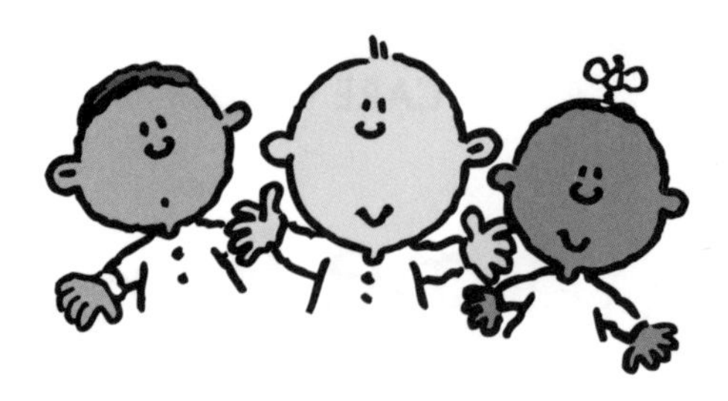

"The National Society for the Prevention of Cruelty to Children (NSPCC) has a vision – a society where all children are loved, valued and able to fulfil their potential. The NSPCC is pleased to work with Egmont World Limited on the development of this series of child care guides. We believe that they will help parents and carers better understand children's and babies' needs."

Jim Harding, Chief Executive, NSPCC.

Designer: Dave Murray
Illustrator: Andy Cooke
Editor: Stephanie Sloan
Cover design: Craig Cameron
Front cover photo supplied by Steve Gorton

NSPCC Registered Charity Number: 216401

Published in Great Britain in 2000 by Egmont World Limited,
a division of Egmont Holding Limited,
Deanway Technology Centre, Wilmslow Road, Handforth,
Cheshire, SK9 3FB. Printed in Italy
ISBN 0 7498 4669 0
A catalogue record for this book is available
from the British Library.

First-time parent

by Faye Corlett

Contents

Introduction

Becoming a parent for the first time is a uniquely rewarding experience. You are suddenly responsible for a new human being whose arrival affects your feelings, relationships and lifestyle. This book aims to help you prepare for baby's arrival and come to terms with your emotions in the first difficult weeks. It offers practical advice on coping with problems and, above all, the reassurance and support that every new parent needs.

Note:
The parent quotations used in this book are taken from the author's experiences working with first-time parents.

When referring to the child, we have alternated the use of he and she throughout the book.

CHAPTER 1

Parenthood

Mums and dads of all ages will find this a useful guide to overcoming most of the initial bumps and shocks of parenthood. How to feed a baby, bathe him, and cope with the million and one so very different things he will need are all skills that need to be learned.

Being a parent must be one of the most difficult jobs in the world. But remember, *everyone* who has their first baby has to jump in at the deep end. Even if you're an experienced babysitter who has

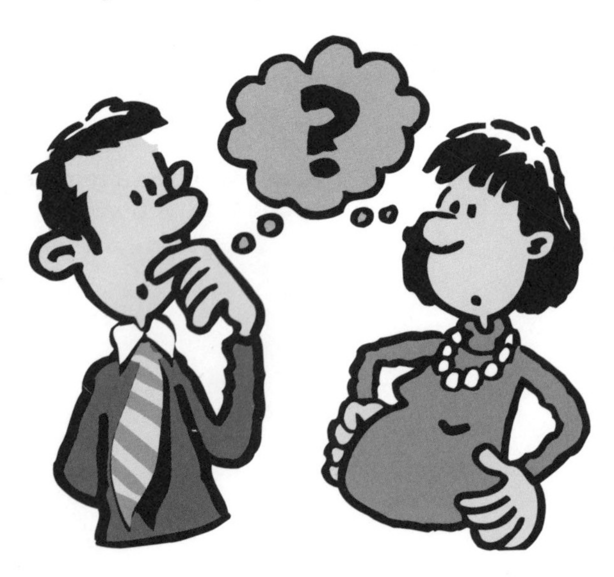

happily dried the tears of hundreds of babies, bringing up your own is guaranteed to be a completely different experience. Because that new little person will be relying on you for all its needs. You will be responsible for a new human being.

Scared? That's a natural emotion to welcome the unknown. You're bound to experience a flood of feelings, some of wonder and joy, others of confusion, of feeling overwhelmed and wondering if you will ever be able to measure up to the needs of a new baby. But every new parent can find reassurance in the fact that, although the prospect may seem scary, being a parent is also one of the most rewarding jobs in the world. That's for certain. Their baby's first smile, first word, first steps, will be a miracles to every parent.

You'll soon find out that you learn pretty fast to survive on a few hours' sleep, manage to do ten jobs at once, and make important decisions about your baby's care. It will be fun, exciting and emotional – just take one day at a time and you'll soon be wondering where baby's first enchanting years have gone!

It's normal too for first-time parents to worry about the pregnancy. Will baby be OK, will there be any problems with the birth? And when thoughts such as that are playing on your mind, those nine months can seem like an awfully long time to wait. Although lots of women find pregnancy a happy time, it can also play havoc with your hormones, and sad times, tearfulness and irritability will make you feel like you're having a personality transplant! Don't worry – the same feelings are being experienced by mums-to-be all over the world.

This book will help you come to terms with your emotions about your new arrival, and help you to realise that whatever you are feeling is normal. It aims to offer advice and tips on:

- preparing for baby's arrival, from what to buy, to making your home safe;
- how to cope with the changes being a parent will bring to your lifestyle;
- tips for single mums, and working mums;
- what to expect in the first few days of caring for your baby;
- what to do when you feel you're not coping, and where to ask for help.

Because being a first-time parent isn't just going to affect your emotions, whether you're the mum or the dad. It's also going to affect every single part of your world. From your home life to your working life, your finances, your relationships, how you plan for the future. From now on, there are going to be at least two of you to think about and consider.

Be prepared. Accept that there will be bad days. Too many tears, sleepless nights, problems with feeding, toilet training – every parent will have them and you will be no exception. Accept too that your bond between you and your baby will be so strong that none of these things will matter when baby smiles and reaches for you or says his first word. These are the true and unique rewards of parenthood.

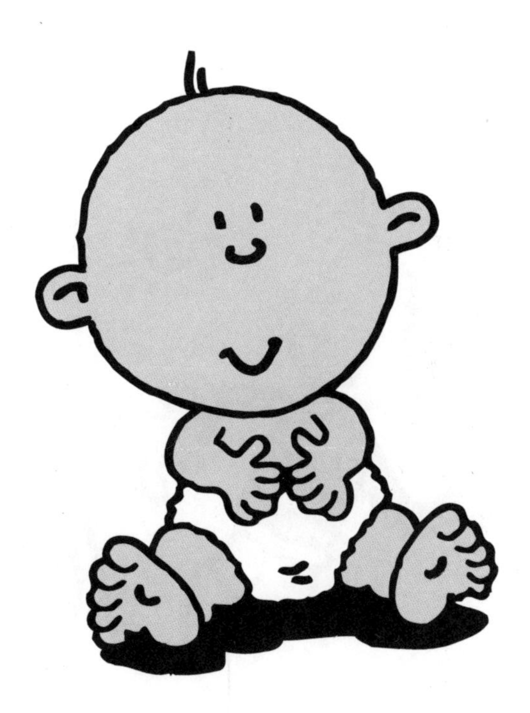

CHAPTER 2

Lifestyle changes

"Before I had Connor, I worked full-time and had a very active social life. Parties, eating out with friends, going to clubs. Now I'm so tired all the time that I don't think I'd even have the energy to get myself ready to go out. But, on the other hand, I feel so happy and proud of him that it really doesn't matter at the moment." (Rachel)

"I used to play football every weekend, and keep myself trim by visiting the local gym a least twice a week. She's (the baby) so tiny though that I've

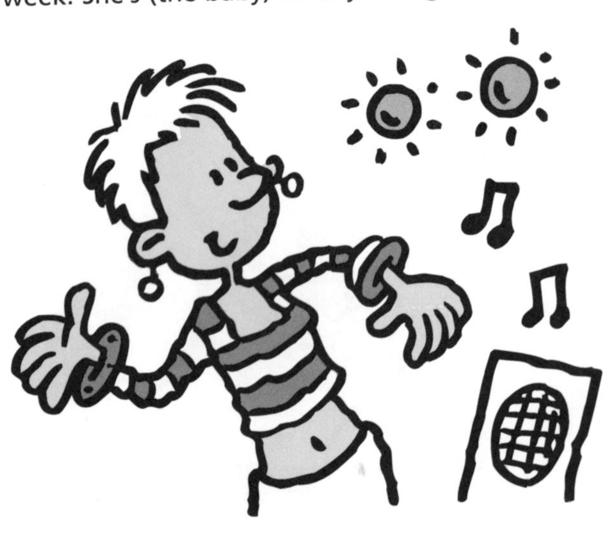

hardly left the house without them for the past two weeks. Lucy (his wife) doesn't say that I can't go training, but I just feel that I've got to be there for both of them." (Marcus)

These first-time parents say it all. When you've got a baby in the house your whole world is turned upside down, because that new infant is reliant on you for his or her every need, 24 hours a day, every day. Even if you are a working parent, you still need to make arrangements for your baby. She is now the centre of your world around which everything else revolves.

A new baby has lots of needs. There will be no mistaking when baby is hungry. She will be quite sure to let you know, as loudly as possible! Babies don't keep to sensible mealtime hours like 12 o'clock or 5 o'clock either. Mums and dads will tell you in unison that babies are very partial to midnight snacks and 3am snacks too!

First-time parents can guarantee that their new baby will be a constant drain on their physical and emotional resources. There will be so many items to buy – nappies, clothes, toys – that even if your social life hasn't disappeared through having to cope with sleepless nights, you may find that money may be too tight to allow you any form of entertainment other than the television.

Perhaps the greatest change comes from having to cope with the rest of your life while at the same time having to cope with a baby. "I've often spent hours just trying to get one job done, but ended the day in frustration without even having started it. Connor would wake up, want his nappy changing, need a feed. It's just constant demands on you." (Rachel)

Tips to help you cope with your new lifestyle

- Try to eat a healthy balanced diet. Remember to drink plenty of water and fruit juice too, especially if you're breastfeeding. You'll be short on time, and often too tired to cook much, but there are lots of healthy fibre and protein-rich foods that will give you the energy to cope. For example, baked beans, baked potatoes, pasta,

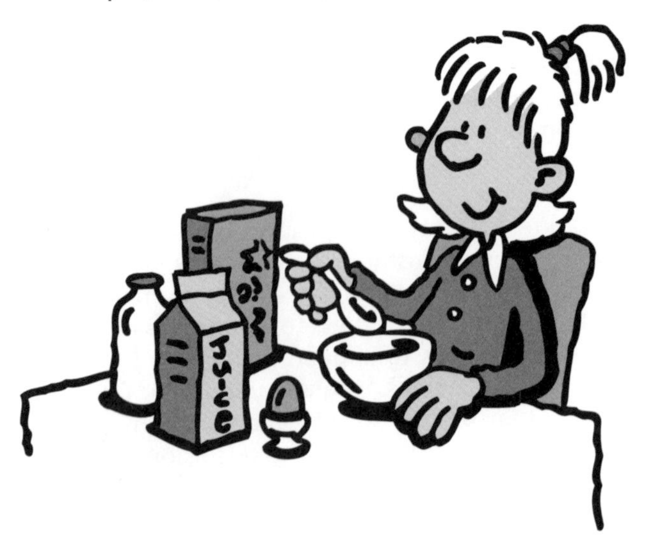

fruit and vegetables, wholegrain breakfast cereals, frozen fish and nuts. These foods are usually quite cheap to buy too.

- Don't expect too much of yourself.
- Don't expect your body to return to normal overnight! Remember, it took nine months to make your baby, so give yourself at least that to get back into shape again.
- Sleep when your baby sleeps, or arrange for a relative or friend to take your baby for a while so you can catch up on your sleep. Share getting up in the night with your partner. Learn a relaxation technique – your local library may have books, tapes or information on this.
- Try to see friends and family. Talk to them about how you feel. Don't be afraid to ask for help, and do accept help when it's offered.
- Make time just for you, even just half an hour relaxing in the bath or reading. Remember you have needs too.

CHAPTER 3

Preparing for baby's arrival

Buying for baby is one of the happiest activities for all first-time parents. Choosing tiny clothes and preparing a nursery will seem to bring the time of birth nearer. Unfortunately, shopping for baby clothes and equipment can be a very expensive business – just ask any of your friends with babies! So that it won't seem quite so costly, start thinking about what you are going to need for your baby early on in the pregnancy, then spread the expenditure over the coming months. Don't be too proud to accept offers of second-hand baby clothes and equipment – some you will only need for a few weeks - so it makes economic sense during what can be a very expensive time!

Essential basics

This is just an idea of the sort of things you will need. At the back of this book you'll find a useful checklist of essential items you can refer to as you shop.

- A selection of sleepsuits or 'babygros' that can be worn day or night, bodysuits, vests, sweaters, socks, fabric booties, hats, mittens, bibs, and for when it's cold outdoors, a warm padded or knitted jacket or bodysuit.
- Nappies, a changing mat, a changing bag, and a

bin for used nappies. The majority of parents prefer the convenience of disposable nappies, but as babies usually need changing around 2,000 times in the first 12 months, these can prove expensive. Terry nappies can be washed, sterilised and used again and again. You will need to weigh up the pros and cons of each against your own budget.

- A baby bath.
- A cot, mattress, blankets and baby bedding. Don't use pillows or duvets as these are dangerous for new-born babies. A second-hand cot is fine, but buy a new mattress which conforms to current safety standards. Make sure it snugly fits the cot so that there is no gap between mattress and frame where your baby

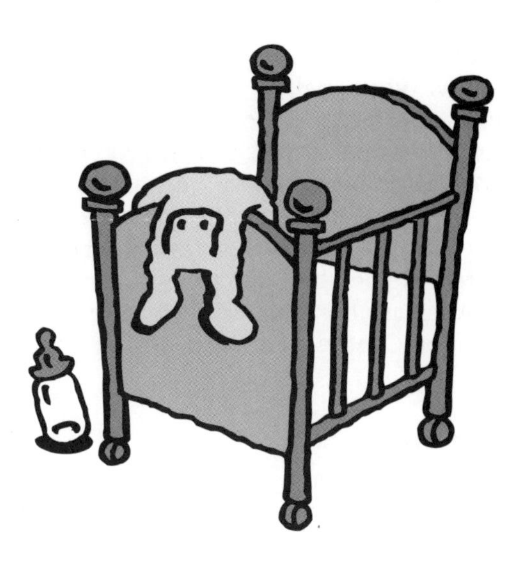

could trap an arm or leg.

- A newborn pram or buggy, and a car seat. A car seat *must* be bought new – don't be tempted to buy second-hand as it may be damaged and vital instructions may be missing. Always have safety uppermost in your mind when choosing equipment to carry and transport your baby. Have a look in your local library for *Which?*, a consumer magazine, which lists the best buys.
- Formula milk and feeding bottles with a bottle steriliser unit, or if you are going to breastfeed your baby, nursing bras and breast pads.
- A medicine chest, with a first-aid kit, baby paracetamol/Calpol, a thermometer and nappy-rash cream.

For first clothes, look for those that are comfortable and cosy, made of soft, natural fabrics that allow your baby's skin to breathe and minimise allergic skin reactions. For first-time parents, it's normal at first to feel awkward about handling your baby, so chose clothes that you can put on and take off with the minimum of fuss. Always check that buttons or fastenings are sewn on securely. Remember, don't buy too many new-born clothes as your baby will all too soon grow out of them. Choose items that are on the larger side.

Safety in the home

Before bringing your baby home, it is also very important that you have a good look around to make sure that you are bringing him into an environment that's as safe as possible. When doing this, remember your baby will all too soon become a toddler, who will happily want to investigate every nook and cranny!

Every year, over half a million children under the age of five go to hospital because of an accident in the home. Be safe rather than sorry and make time to follow these basic safety steps before baby arrives:

- Make sure rugs and carpets are firmly fitted to the floor;
- Guard open and electric fires;
- Fit plug and socket guards and check for any frayed or hanging flexes such as the kettle flex, that could electrocute or injure your baby;
- If you have stairs, fit a child safety gate to avoid tumbles;
- Make drawers and cupboards baby-proof by fitting safety catches and finger-trap guards to doors;
- If you don't have a smoke alarm, get one fitted. This is an essential safety measure for the whole family;
- Ensure items such as bleach, medicines and any equipment liable to cause injury, such as kitchen knives or glasses, are stored well out of your baby's reach.

Most importantly, when you bring your baby

home, *don't* leave him unattended. When he's sleeping in his cot, check on him periodically.

Your health visitor should be able to give you more information on how to prevent accidents in the home. Or contact *The Child Accident Prevention Trust* who will be able to provide common-sense help and advice on child safety (see Chapter 11: When you need help, for their full details).

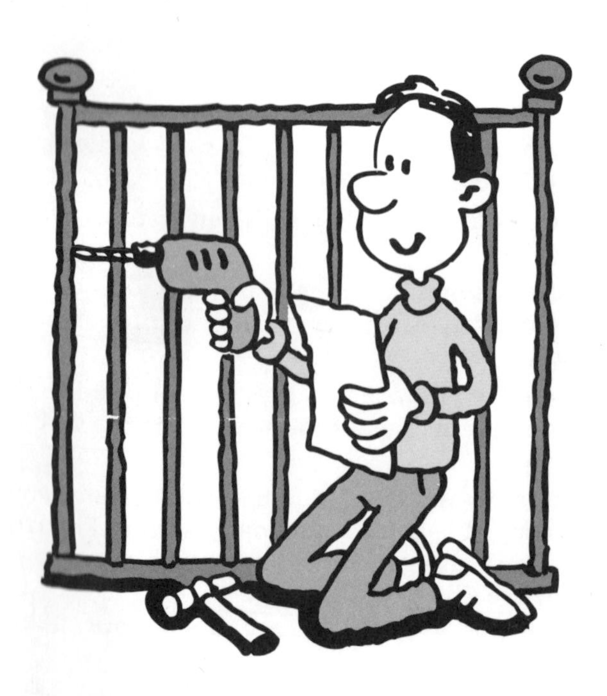

CHAPTER 4

First days at home

Congratulations on being a first-time parent! You've brought your new baby home and an exciting chapter in life is about to start for all the family.

Holding your baby

You will probably feel all fingers and thumbs about lifting and cuddling your baby at first. There's no need to be worried because babies are much stronger than they appear.

- Place one hand under her neck and head and slip your other arm under baby's back. The head can then be easily cradled inside your elbow whilst you support the bottom with your hand. Hold your baby close to your body.
- A baby's neck muscles take a few weeks to grow strong so make sure you ALWAYS support the head of your newborn.
- For safety, always put your baby down on her back, bringing the body down first and supporting the head until it touches the cot mattress.

Nappy changing

Get ready for around 8 to 12 nappy changes every day in your baby's first weeks! To keep your baby's bottom dry and avoid soreness and nappy rash, you will also need to clean her bottom after each change. The secret to easy nappy changing is organisation. First, gather the things you need together – nappy, changing mat, warm water and cotton wool or baby wipes, tissues for drying and a nappy bin for the dirty nappy and wipes.

- Always change baby's nappy on a flat surface. The floor is best. If you use a changing unit or the bed, make sure the baby doesn't roll off. Never leave the baby unattended.
- To prevent germs, always clean a baby girl's bottom from front to back, and make sure to dry well all around.

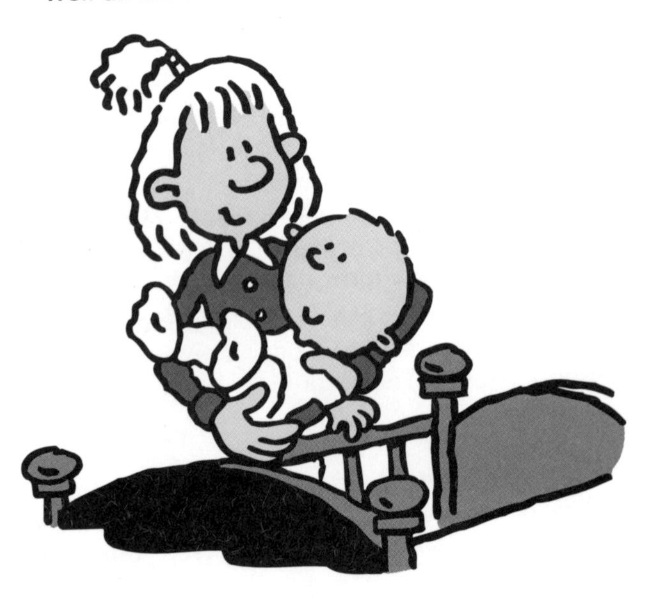

- Disposable nappies are easy to put on and are fastened by sticky tabs. Terry nappies need to be folded into an upside-down triangle, with the three corners fastened at the front by a nappy pin. Make sure the nappy fits baby's bottom snugly but not too tightly.

Bathing baby

This is probably one of the most daunting tasks for first-time parents. As long as you hold baby securely following the tips given below, you will manage just fine.

- Ask a midwife to help you the first time you bath your baby.
- Use a baby bath. Only half fill the baby bath with warm water and always check the temperature with your elbow first. When bathing baby, always support the head and neck with one hand whilst you wash with the other. It will help to make your baby feel secure if you smile and talk too, making bathtime a fun time for both of you.
- Try not to get water into your baby's eyes and use only a small amount of baby soap to prevent drying up her skin. To dry baby, lay her down on top of a towel on the floor. Dry her carefully and gently with a soft towel.

Don't overdo it!

If you planned to quickly get into a daily routine with your new baby, you'll soon realise that you might as well tear up those plans! Even with a crystal ball you won't be able to predict when baby will sleep, wake up, cry, or need feeding and changing. No two days will be the same. Be prepared for the fact that it will all seem a bit chaotic at first. It might take you hours just to get yourself and your baby dressed in the morning – this is quite normal! It'll be best for you to let your baby take the lead.

- Take a nap when baby naps.
- Snack on healthy foods, with plenty of fresh fruit and vegetables.
- Try not to worry about the housework – tomorrow's another day.

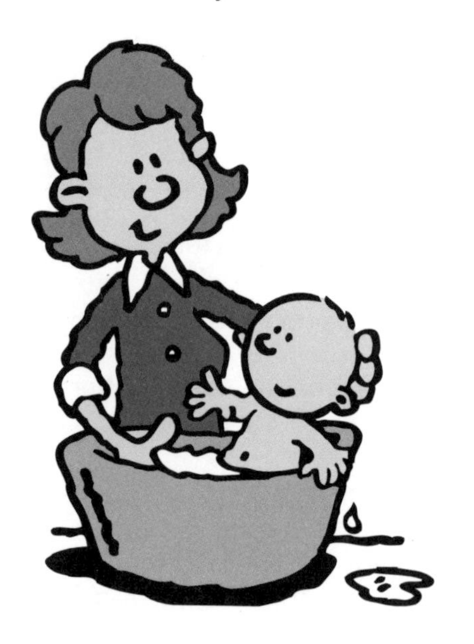

- Ask for help, and accept help when it's offered.

Although mums often feel they have to accept the largest part of caring for the new arrival, they should encourage and allow dads to take control sometimes. Share all the baby jobs and chores as much as possible. Remember, baby and dad will also benefit as it will help in forming a bond between them.

You have to accept that, now you're parents, life will never be the same again. You can make it work for all the family by taking each day as it comes and not expecting too much of yourselves in the early days.

CHAPTER 5

Bonding

While getting ready for being a parent, you may have heard of or read the words "bond" and "bonding" as being about the special relationship between a mum and her baby just after the birth. But although this is a big part of the bonding process, bonding is much more than just that. It's a shared feeling of togetherness, love and security between both parents and their baby that brings emotional fulfilment to everyone in the family.

When you bond with your baby you form a deep and mutual attachment. You will soon learn to

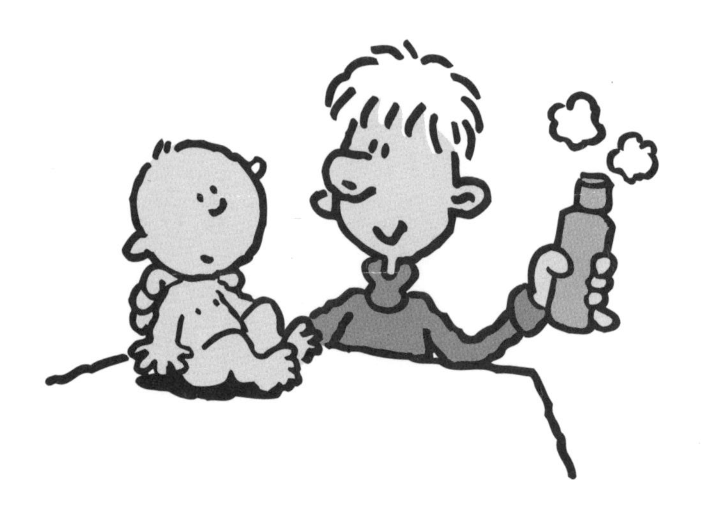

distinguish different 'types' of cry and what they mean your baby needs - a cuddle, a nappy change, a feed, and so on. A secure bond between parents and baby will help the baby see relationships as comforting and reassuring, giving it a promising start to a healthy life emotionally.

Bonding starts with love for your baby. This can begin even during pregnancy, and both parents can take an active role in starting to develop early on what is a very special part of the parent and child relationship. It can be as simple as taking turns to softly rub mum's stomach when she's relaxing and feeling the baby's movements. Yes, the baby is able to hear your voice in the womb, so gently talk to the 'bump' and think of it as a real person, which will strengthen your future bond. During the pregnancy you'll more than likely have quiet times together talking about the baby, perhaps discussing names or colours for a nursery, and these are ideal opportunities to begin baby bonding.

It is true that, for most mums, immediately after the baby's birth is the time when the strongest bond is formed between mum and baby. This is partly because the emotions surrounding the birth open the way for strong feelings towards the new-born. Immediately after birth mums also start to produce a hormone called 'prolactin'. This is linked to the production of breast milk, and so helps to stimulate 'mothering' feelings towards the baby. Studies have shown that most mums behave in the same way when they first hold their baby. They look into their baby's eyes and feel all the fingers and toes as they say their first words to the new infant. And because newborns can smell, taste, hear and see, so the smell of their mum, the warmth of her body and the sound of her heartbeat will make the baby feel comforted and secure.

But this is really only *one* possible time for beginning to feel love for your baby. Giving birth is a tiring experience, and for some, a difficult birth and the effects of medication during labour can affect how you feel when you see your baby. Women can also react differently to the special

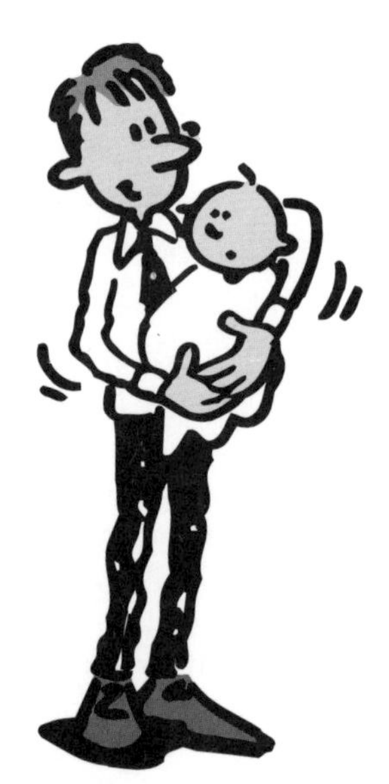

hormones produced during the birth. So don't worry if bonding takes time. It's not a once and only event but a growing feeling that develops as you and baby get to know each other. Neither will the bond be reduced if your baby is born by Caesarean and you are unable to hold him immediately after birth, or if he needs special care in a baby incubator. Even for those who miss out on early contact, the bond that develops will be just as strong.

Bonding with the family

The bond between a mum and her baby is perhaps more instinctive, probably because she's carried the baby and is usually the first one to give baby a cuddle after the birth. But a dad who is encouraged right from the beginning to share in baby's care can form just as strong a bond as a mum can. And it is important for baby's future development that he is given the opportunity to form bonds with all members of the family. So be sure that dad gets involved – changing nappies, bathing baby, feeding, cuddling, every part of baby's care. The more time a dad can spend with baby, the stronger their bond will become.

Useful tips

You can help to make a lasting and secure bond with your baby by:

- Helping to create a bond even before your baby is born by seeing your 'bump' as a real person, talking to it and sharing your life with it;

- Making time for plenty of loving cuddles with your baby so he learns to recognise you as a parent and someone to be relied on for his needs;
- Making eye contact with your baby and talking to him – although he may be too young to understand exactly what you are saying, he will enjoy listening to your voice and will soon learn to respond in his own way;
- Encouraging bonding in the family and with other people close to you by involving them in the care of your baby as much as possible;
- Not leaving your baby to cry. It is baby's only way of communicating with you. He may need changing, he may be hungry or just in need of a cuddle. See Chapter 10: Problems, for advice on what to do when your baby cries.

CHAPTER 6

Family relationships

As your whole lifestyle changes as a first-time parent, so will your relationships, especially with your partner. Athough parent roles have changed a great deal over the past thirty years and many dads do stay at home to look after the baby, generally it is the mum who takes on this role. And if she is breastfeeding this can mean little time to herself. If dad is working, he might feel under more pressure to work harder for his new little family. At the end of the day, he comes home to a crying baby and a tired partner who may be just beginning to feel a little resentful about how

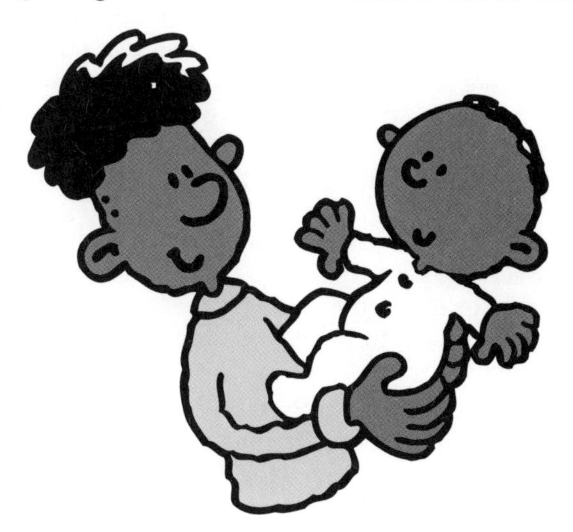

much her life has changed. This can make for a strained relationship, in which the couple begin to wonder if they will ever be on the same footing again!

Even the best of relationships are often strained by parenthood. This is mainly because you will have less time to spend with each other, to share joint interests, or time just to talk. But while a new mum might feel resentful because she is the one who normally bears the greatest burden of care, a new dad can often feel left out because the baby is taking up so much of his partner's attention.

From the moment she brings her first baby home, mum should try to make dad feel included. He needs to feel that he is needed and is participating in the baby's care, and isn't just an observer. Making sure he takes an active role will not only help share the burden but is also important in helping him to forge his own very special relationship with the baby. Couples should try if possible to share their responsibilities for the baby.

- However close you were before the birth, don't expect your partner to be able to read your mind. Let each other know if there is a problem and find time to share your feelings with your partner.
- Make time for each other. Even if it's only a trip to the shops or a walk in the park, ask a friend or relative to look after baby for a short time so that you can be together.

- Go to bed together, early if you can. Spend the time relaxing and take it as an opportunity to talk about your day.
- Share caring for the baby and household chores as much as possible.

Sex is part of any normal secure relationship, but you might find that having a baby in the home doesn't always make for an easy sex life. Caring for your first baby is tiring and the demands the baby makes on your time will also mean that opportunities for sex with your partner may be limited. It doesn't help the situation that many women will also feel uncomfortable and sore for some weeks after the birth so that sex with their

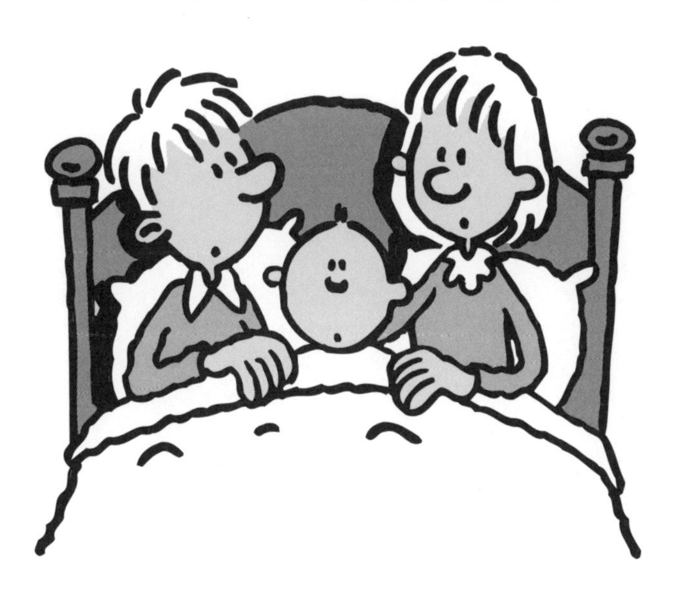

partner is the last thing on their minds.

- Find the time for plenty of cuddles instead so that you still feel close to each other;
- Don't rush to get things back to normal. Listen to each other, talk about your feelings and realise that a successful relationship needs to be worked at all the time;
- If sex is painful, tell your partner, and take things easy at first. If you are worried about the pain, see your family doctor.

Finally, being first-time parents is an important time to maintain your sense of humour! If you can laugh off any problems in your relationship you'll soon find out that, wonder of wonders, the baby has brought you closer together after all!

CHAPTER 7

Single mum

People often assume that if you are having a baby, you're part of a relationship and will have a partner to share in bringing up your new infant. Increasingly today, mums are bringing up their baby alone. In fact, around one in five families is now headed by a single parent, and in the majority of those cases, that parent is the mum.

Being a single mum is bound to reduce the number of choices you have in deciding how to bring up your baby. You may want to work but perhaps the job you do will not bring in enough money to cover childminder or crèche fees.

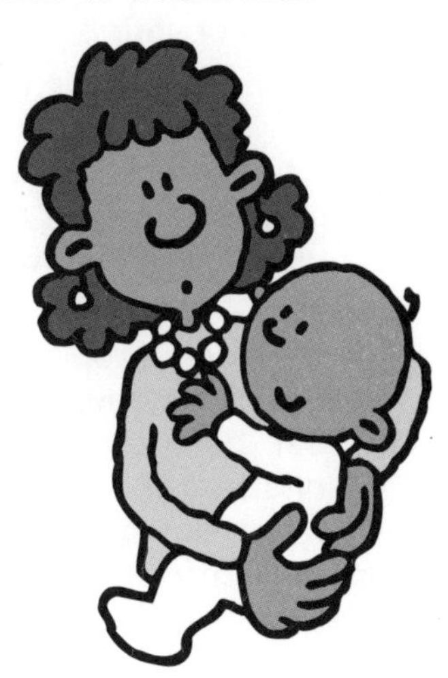

It is normal even for mums who are in a relationship to feel lonely and isolated staying at home with the baby, and getting out to see people can seem like a huge task. As one new single mum says, "I worked before so I had people to talk to. Now there's only her (the baby) most of the time. I think it's made me withdrawn, you know, no confidence, and I'm even shy speaking to people in the shops."

- If you have family members nearby, accept their offers of help and support as often as possible. Although you will feel you have a lot on your plate just caring for your baby, keep in touch with friends, and make sure you see them from time to time. Keeping in touch with the people you know you can count on will mean that there is support there for you during a crisis, for example, if ever you or your baby is ill.
- If you don't know people in the local area, your hospital maternity unit or your health visitor should be able to tell you about mother and baby groups. These are excellent places to get to know other .people, and you will all have something in common – a baby!
- Sometimes the demands of coping single-handed can overwhelm a single mum, but thankfully there is a great deal of professional help available. Organisations like *Gingerbread*, a self-help association for one-parent families, have local groups who offer support, friendship, information, advice and practical help. Look

under Chapter 11: When you need help for how to contact *Gingerbread*.

Unless you really need to keep your partner away, perhaps if he is abusive, it will help with your baby's development if you are able to let him see the baby regularly. Naturally, if you hoped to be bringing up your baby as part of a couple, you might have angry feelings towards the baby's father. Try to remember that these feelings are your own, not your baby's, and allow as much access as you can. If you stay on friendly terms with him, he may even help with minding the baby, giving you some important free time when you can socialise or catch up on your sleep.

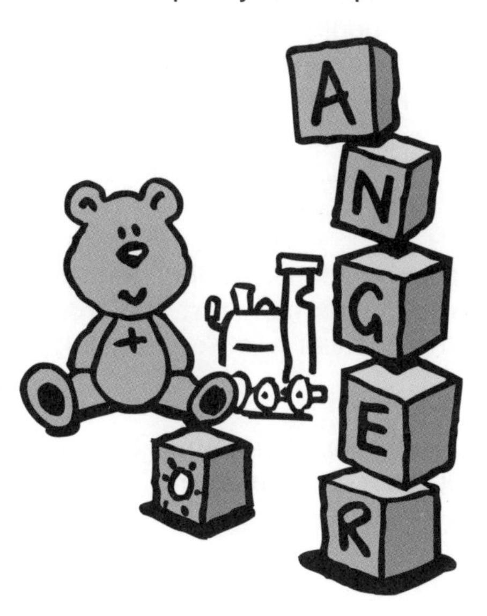

Another major headache for single mums can be money. Even if you have a well-paid job and intend to carry on working, there'll be so many things the baby needs – clothes, nappies, toiletries – you'll wonder where all your money goes. It's important, therefore to find out about all the benefits that are available for single-parent families so that you can claim all you are entitled to.

- Visit your local Benefits Agency Office (you'll find the address in your phone book) for information on entitlements and help with making claims.
- Other useful sources of information are your local Citizens Advice Bureau and the Department of Social Services (again, the addresses will be in your phone book under Citizens Advice, and under your local County Council).
- If you need help with claiming maintenance from the baby's father, contact the Child Support Agency helpline on 0345 133133 (local call charge).

Don't feel proud about claiming. Remember that you are putting your baby first and ensuring that you have the finances to make life work for both of you.

Do feel proud about your great achievement in bringing up baby on your own. This is no mean task. As a single mum, you will also have the reward of developing a unique relationship with your baby.

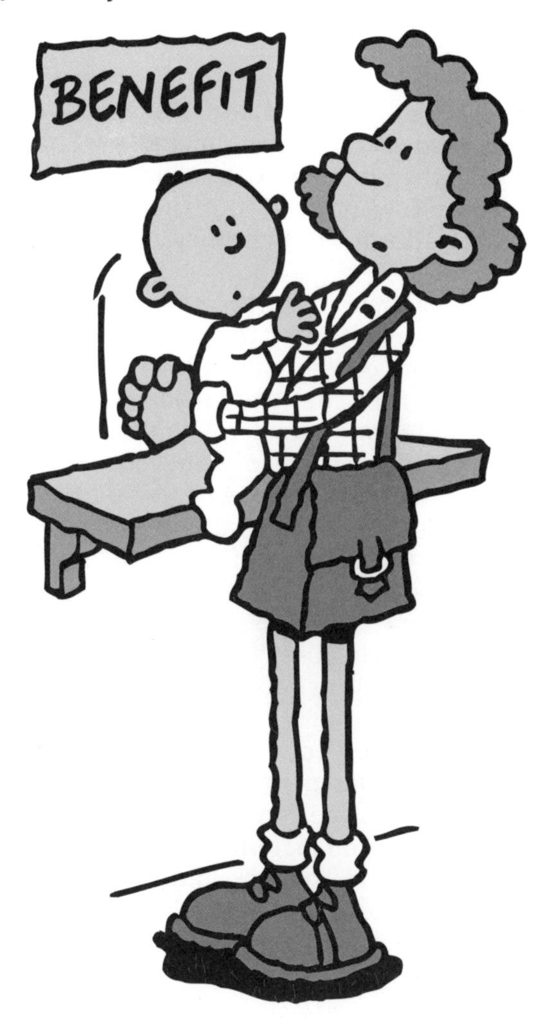

CHAPTER 8

Working mum

Helped by new government standards and improved childcare provision, mums now have more choice when it comes to deciding whether or not to work. Nowadays, 45% of new mums go back to work after the birth of their baby.

There are many important reasons why you as a first-time mum might want to continue working. Yours may be the only income if you are a single mum or your partner has been made redundant; you may be following a career; you may want to work to give you a sense of value; or perhaps because your own mother coped successfully with work and children. If you have always worked, you may also have to ask yourself if you would feel right about being dependent on your partner financially. Work can also give you another outlook on life – because staying at home with baby can often feel very isolating for some mums.

- Make sure you tell your employer as soon as possible about your pregnancy. Employers are legally required to keep a woman's job open for her if she is going on maternity leave. If you are intending to return to work, discuss with your employer the opportunities for working part-time on your return. Or perhaps job-sharing (equally sharing your current hours with a colleague), or working more family-friendly, flexible hours (coming into work later and leaving earlier) may be possible. Sorting things out during your pregnancy will not only give your employer time to make new arrangements to help you. It will also enable you to organise good childcare where your baby will be loved and well cared for;

- There is a standard entitlement for maternity leave. In general, every woman who is in work while she is pregnant is entitled to at least 18 weeks' maternity leave. Maternity pay depends very much upon your individual circumstances regarding length of service with your employer and your National Insurance contributions. Check your details first with your employer. If

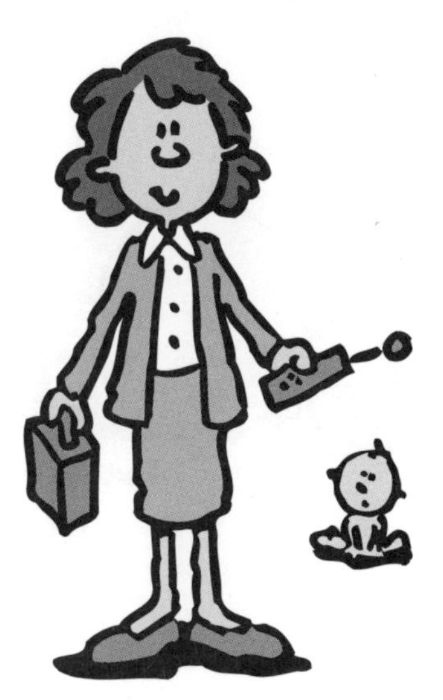

you need any further help, contact your local Benefits Agency Office (you'll find the address in your phone book) who will be able to work out your entitlements based on your personal situation.

Whatever your reasons for working, you are bound to experience mixed emotions about leaving your new baby when the time comes. It is normal to worry that your baby will not be happy without you, or that his or her development will be affected because you are not there.

- A common worry is that your baby may feel more love for the person who cares for them while you are at work.
- You might also worry that your baby won't be cared for properly.

Childcare

The secret to any working mum's success and the way to make these worries disappear is organisation. If you make carefully planned childcare arrangements that you are content with and are satisfied that your baby is being well cared for, this is sure to give you much more confidence about going out to work.

Options for childcare include:

- A family member or close friend. Perhaps you have a close relative, such as your mum or mum-in-law, or a trusted family friend with good experience of caring for her own children who is at home during the day and who could care for your baby;
- A day nursery or crèche. These are either privately run (and must be council registered) or under the control of your local council. Perhaps your workplace has its own day nursery or crèche. Using this facility can give you the opportunity to see your baby during the day, and you will also be nearby in case of illness or emergency. You will be able to find details of day nurseries and crèches in your area from your council social services department;
- A childminder. Childminders are usually mums themselves who care for children in their own homes. Anyone paid to look after children under five in this way must apply to register with the council social services department, who check

the person's suitability and that they can give a good standard of care;

- A nanny. A child's nanny is someone who generally 'lives in', that is, shares your home and facilities. As nannies don't have to be registered with the local council, it is very important you check that they have excellent personal references and are qualified to care for your baby. Recognised qualifications in childcare include the Diploma in Nursery Nursing (formerly the NNEB qualification), NVQ in Childcare and BTEC National Diploma in Childhood Studies;
- Whatever option you choose, remember that it is important to only entrust the care of your baby to a loving person who will look after your baby well. Before you make a decision on childcare for your baby, ask for recommendations from other parents. Visit a shortlist of care providers. Ask questions and go with your instincts – it's a good sign if you like the feel of the place and the children there seem safe and happy.

Below is a useful list of questions to ask when considering childcare in day nurseries/crèches and with childminders. Jot them down to take with you when visiting possible baby-care providers. Then you can compare the responses and choose the best option for your baby.

Choosing childcare – questions to ask

- Is the childminder, day nursery/crèche registered with the local council? Ask to see their certificate of registration.

- What is the ratio of staff to babies/ children?
- Are the staff qualified to care for children? Recognised qualifications include the Diploma in Nursery Nursing (or NNEB), NVQ in Childcare, and BTEC National Diploma in Childhood Studies.
- What facilities are there, such as equipment, space to play?
- What sort of discipline is used?
- What would my baby's day be like?

Make sure you explain your baby's special needs to your childminder or crèche staff, for example, feeding information and likes and dislikes. It is also especially important that they know about any

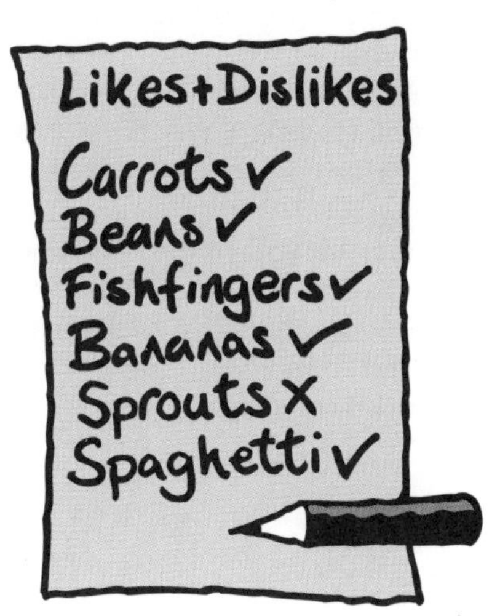

health problems your baby may have. Most importantly, always leave a name and contact number with whoever is minding your baby so you can be quickly reached in an emergency.

When you are home, try to forget about work and make the most of the time you have together. Make baby's bathtimes and feeding times special occasions for the whole family. Plan ahead to book odd days off work so that you can spend all day with your baby. If you can have quality time with your baby when you are at home, there is no reason at all why being a working mum should have a bad effect on your unique relationship.

To make going back to work easier, stay in touch with colleagues while you are on maternity leave so they can keep you up to date with work news. Ask if it will be possible to return to work gradually, perhaps doing two or three days a week for the first month, which will help you to see if your childcare arrangements are working out.

As a first-time parent you cannot pretend that you only have yourself to please. But remember that you are also high up on the list of priorities in your new family. The important thing is to find a balance that is right for you.

CHAPTER 9

The baby blues

Becoming a parent is certainly a wonderful experience. Feelings of pride and happiness are generally uppermost at the birth. But for some mums, these feelings are replaced by topsy-turvy emotions that they find hard to explain when they suffer from the 'baby blues'.

About half of all mums feel sad and blue after giving birth. Common symptoms include bursting into tears for no real reason, and feeling exhausted yet unable to sleep. Experts believe these feelings are due to the sweeping hormonal changes caused by pregnancy joined with a mix of emotions about the birth. You will feel great happiness about bringing a new life into the world, yet anxious that everything will turn out right.

As one new mum says, "I expected to be crying after the birth, but I thought they would be tears of joy. Everything just felt as if it had been turned upside down and I was thinking straight away that I couldn't cope. But it passed. And after talking to other mums, I realised it was normal to feel like that."

So try not to worry if you experience the baby blues. Difficult as it may be, tell yourself that they are normal after pregnancy and delivery. For the majority of mums, they soon disappear and you can help them fade away quickly by being prepared for the experience beforehand. Explain to your partner that it is normal for mums to feel low after their baby is born. They can then be prepared to give you the help and support you need, and jointly share in caring for the baby. Dads in turn should remember to be understanding; telling your partner to "pull yourself together" is not a solution. Make sure she gets plenty of rest, and plenty of cuddles from you.

To keep the blues from taking over your life and spoiling your enjoyment of your new baby, avoid expecting too much of yourself in the first weeks

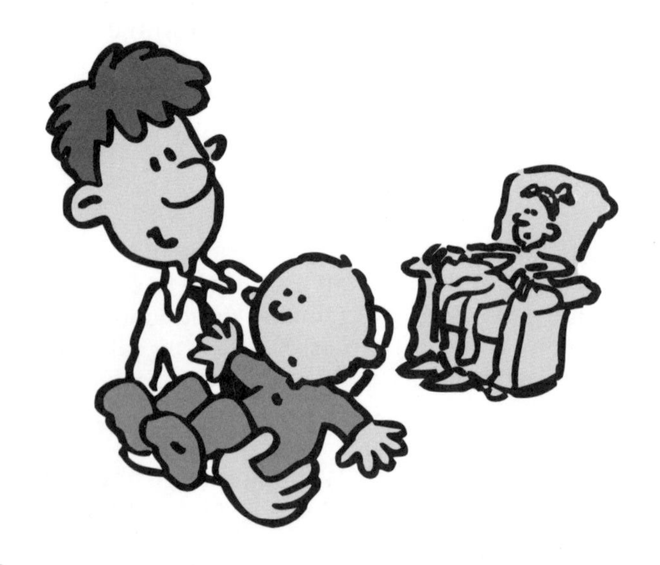

after the birth. Ask for and accept help when it's offered, but limit visitors (and the number of visits!) just to those people you feel comfortable with. Don't feel obliged to entertain people with your new baby. Be prepared too for 'helpful' comments, especially from your mum or mum-in-law who "did things differently in my day."

Although having the baby blues is normal, it's important to seek help straight away if they appear to last for some time after the birth of your baby. This is because you may be suffering from post-natal depression. Post-natal depression is completely different from the baby blues. Although some of the symptoms may be the same – crying, feeling exhausted – post-natal depression is more than just feeling unhappy for a short time. It's when you feel hopeless and unable to cope at all.

If you recognise all or some of these feelings that carry on or suddenly appear well after the birth of your baby:

- you're tired, but you can't sleep;
- you have no interest in either your baby or yourself;
- you find even the smallest tasks just impossible;
- you just can't stop crying.

Seek help as soon as possible. This kind of depression is an illness so it is very important both for yourself and your family that you get some help. Even though you might find it a real effort to talk about your feelings, do try to overcome this hurdle. Speak to your doctor or health visitor. You'll almost certainly find that talking things through with someone who knows how you are feeling will make things much better. There are also a number of support groups who will be only too pleased to share your problems. Look under Chapter 11: When you need help, for the details of *MAMA (Meet-a-Mum Association)* and *Parentline*, for just two of the organisations available.

Post-natal depression is an illness that can be successfully treated. Support, and sometimes medication, will often make a big difference – it's never too late to seek help!

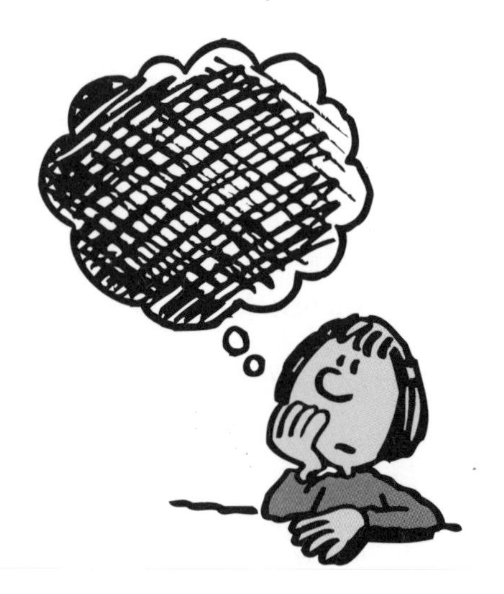

CHAPTER 10

Problems

All first-time parents will be anxious about the health and well-being of their newborn baby. Especially in the first few weeks when everything is strange, it is often hard to know what is normal and when you can be confident that nothing is wrong with your baby. It is quite natural for you to worry about why the baby is crying, for example, or why she won't sleep, or to question that she is ill. In bonding with your baby, you will gradually get to know her different cries and how to respond – with a feed, a nappy change, or just a cuddle. Remember however, *never hesitate* to seek advice from your doctor or health visitor when you are worried or think your baby is unwell.

Thankfully, more often then not, problems such as prolonged crying or sleeplessness can be solved.

Baby won't stop crying

Babies cry for lots of different reasons at all times of the day, the most common being that they are hungry or thirsty. They also cry because they are tired, too hot or too cold, if they need a nappy change, or from lack of physical contact.

If your baby just won't stop crying, try the following useful tips:

- Picking up your baby often helps. Hold her close and rock her gently in your arms while you quietly talk or sing and walk around. The motion and the sound of your heartbeat will be soothing, and can also help in making baby go off to sleep;
- Change baby's nappy if it needs changing;
- Even if your baby has had a feed, she may still be hungry. Most babies do go through unsettled spells when they demand to be fed frequently. See if she will take a feed from you;
- Your baby might have a touch of 'colic', a kind of stomach cramp, which is normal for young babies. Babies with colic often draw their legs up to their stomach while they cry, and their crying

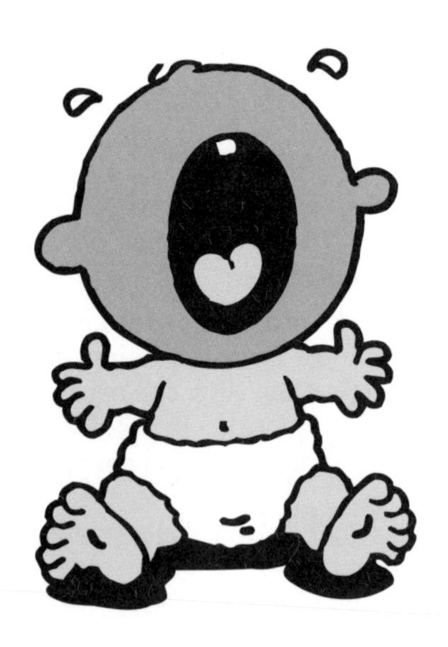

may be irregular – stopping for a moment or two then starting up again. Cuddle and rock your baby as above. If you find that the colic attacks happen regularly, don't hesitate to seek advice from your doctor or health visitor;

- Check your baby's temperature by feeling the back of her neck to see if it feels cold or sweaty. Wrap baby up more securely if she feels cold, and change her clothes or cover her body with a lighter blanket if she feels too warm;
- Fresh air and a change of scene can also work wonders. Try a walk with baby, or take her for a drive. Again, baby will find the motion soothing.

Baby won't sleep

Some babies sleep better than others. Your baby will have her own unique pattern of sleeping and waking, but it's unlikely to be the same as yours! It will help if you encourage sleeping at night from the start by showing your baby that night-time is different from daytime. When feeding your baby at night, keep the light and your voice low. Keep the sociable laughing and play times with your baby for the daylight hours.

As with a crying baby, your baby might not be sleeping because she is hungry or thirsty, needs a nappy change, is too hot or too cold, or just needs a cuddle. Follow the tips above for dealing with these common problems. Also:

- Check the temperature in baby's room. It's just as

important that it isn't too hot as too cold. Try to keep the room temperature at a constant 16 to 20 degrees centigrade.

Symptoms of illness that need urgent attention

The following signs indicate illness in a baby or young child and should *never* be ignored:

- Loss of consciousness;
- A convulsion (fit), or blueness of lips or face;
- A very high temperature. The normal body

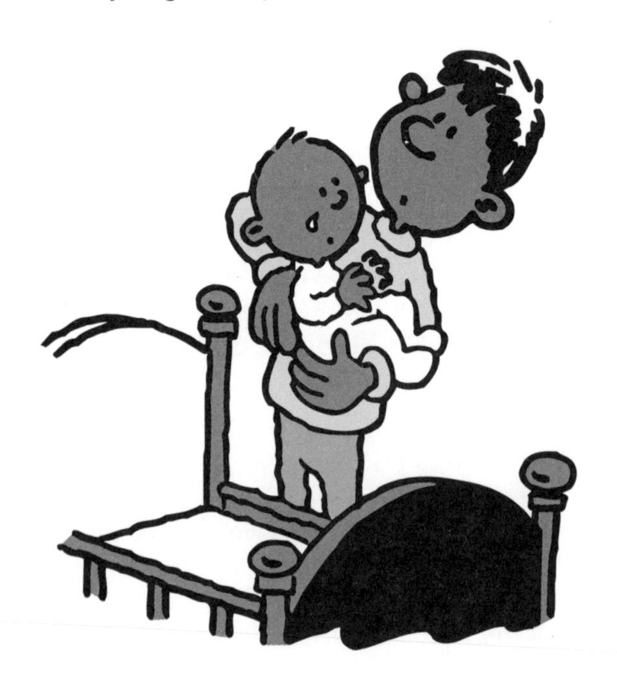

temperature for a child is between 36 and 37 degrees centigrade (97 to 98.6 fahrenheit). To take your baby's temperature, first rinse the thermometer in cold water and then shake it with a flick of the wrist. Make sure it has a low reading. Then place the mercury bulb end under your baby's armpit and hold it in place for two minutes;

- Your baby has a temperature, but her hands and feet feel cold and clammy;
- Breathing difficulties, breathing fast or noisy breathing, which may be combined with a hoarse cough;
- Your baby seems unusually drowsy or hard to wake;
- A rash that looks like bleeding under the skin;
- Persistent vomiting and diarrhoea;
- Crying in an unusual way or for an unusually long time, and seeming to be in a lot of pain;
- Refusing feeds.

Most importantly, trust your instincts. Even as a new parent, you'll know better than anyone what is normal day-to-day behaviour for your baby. If you are at all worried, contact your doctor. Even if it turns out that nothing is wrong with baby, that's fine. Never feel afraid of asking for medical help.

Make a note here of the contact numbers for your doctor and health visitor, and keep this book in a safe place so the numbers are easily accessible when you need them.

DOCTOR Telephone number

....

HEALTH VISITOR Telephone number

....

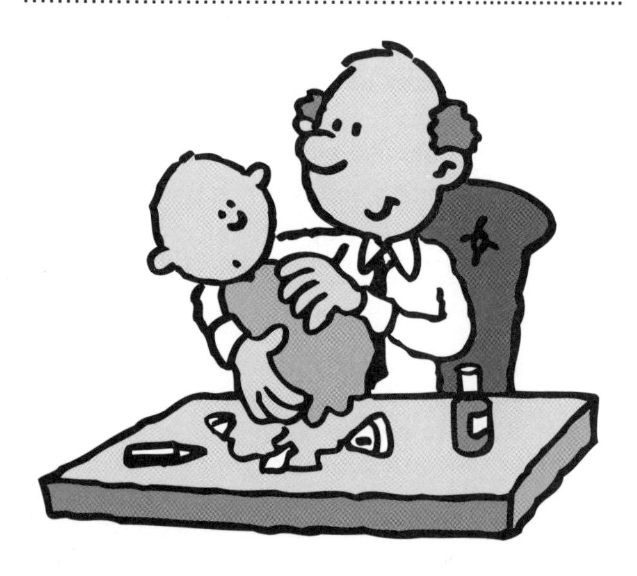

CHAPTER 11

When you need help

The good news for first-time parents is that expert help is often only a telephone call away. There are lots of excellent help groups who know that being a first-timer isn't always easy, perhaps even more so if you're bringing up a baby on your own. Try your own local health visitor, GP, midwife or local health clinic for advice on what help is available near you.

There's certainly a good deal to learn and to experience for all first-time parents. The support groups listed here are used to offering help and encouragement to thousands of parents. So don't ever feel scared or guilty about getting in touch – it won't mean that you are a bad parent. Support is there for you whenever you need it.

Behaviour difficulties

Serene (incorporating the CRY-SIS Helpline)

London WC1N 3XX

Helpline : 020 7404 5011 (8am-11pm)

Provides emotional support and practical advice to parents dealing with excessive crying, demanding behaviour and sleep problems. Callers are put in touch with local volunteers who have had similar experiences.

General support groups

Home-Start UK

2 Salisbury Road, Leicester LE1 7QR
Telephone 0116 233 9955

A voluntary home-visiting support scheme for families with children under five.

National Childbirth Trust (NCT)

Alexandra House, Oldham Terrace,
Acton, London W3 6NH
Telephone 020 8992 8637

Help, support and advice for mothers.

Parentline Plus

Highgate Studios, 53-79 Highgate Road,
Kentish Town, London NW5 1TL
Telephone 0808 800 2222
Textphone (for speech and hearing impaired)
0800 783 6783
www.parentlineplus.org.uk

Incorporates the 'Parentline' freephone helpline which offers support and information for anyone in a parenting role.

Post-natal depression

Association for Post-natal Illness

25 Jerdan Place. London SW6 1BE
Telephone 020 7386 0868

Advice and support for people suffering from post-natal depression.

Meet-A-Mum Association (MAMA)
Waterside Centre, 26 Avenue Road,
South Norwood, London SE25 4DX
Telephone 020 8771 5595

Support for mums suffering from post-natal depression, loneliness and isolation.

Safety

Child Accident Prevention Trust

18-20 Farringdon Lane, London EC1R 3HA
Telephone 020 7608 3828

Help and advice for parents on child safety.

Royal Society for the Prevention of Accidents (RoSPA)

Edgbaston Park, 353 Bristol Road,
Birmingham B5 7ST
Telephone 0121 248 2000

Advice on accident prevention.

Single parents

Gingerbread

16-17 Clerkenwell Close, London EC1R 0AN
Telephone 020 7336 8183

Self-help association for one-parent families.

Working parents

Parents At Work

77 Holloway Road, London N7 8JZ

Telephone 020 7628 2128

Advice and support for working parents.

NSPCC

NSPCC National Centre
42 Curtain Road
London EC2A 3NH
Website: www.nspcc.org.uk

The National Society for the Prevention of Cruelty to Children (NSPCC) is the UK's leading charity specialising in child protection and the prevention of cruelty to children. It also operates the NSPCC Child Protection Helpline – a free, 24 hour service which provides counselling, information and advice to anyone concerned about a child at risk of abuse. The Helpline number is: 0808 800 5000, Textphone: 0800 056 0566.

What to do in a medical emergency

Even though you may do all you can to avoid accidents in the home and to keep your baby healthy, there may come a time when your baby needs urgent medical help.

At times such as these, follow these guidelines:

- Call your doctor. Outside surgery hours, a recorded message will usually tell you how to get in touch with the doctor;

- If you can't get an answer at your doctor's surgery, take your baby to the Accident and Emergency Department of your nearest hospital. As a rule, Accident and Emergency is open 24 hours a day, every day of the year;
- If your baby's condition is life-threatening, don't hesitate in dialling 999 and asking for an ambulance. Tell the operator that it is needed for a baby. If you have to call from a phone box you won't need any change as 999 calls are free.

Conclusion

Being a first-time parent may present its fair share of worry, but it is a uniquely rewarding experience. You are bound to have trying times, especially in the first few weeks when you are adapting to your new lifestyle. You'll probably wonder how someone so small can manage to wreak such havoc on your routine! Persevere – things *will* get better. The early days may be tough, but just take one day at a time. You'll soon be looking back on them with affection and realising just how much you've learned about being a parent.

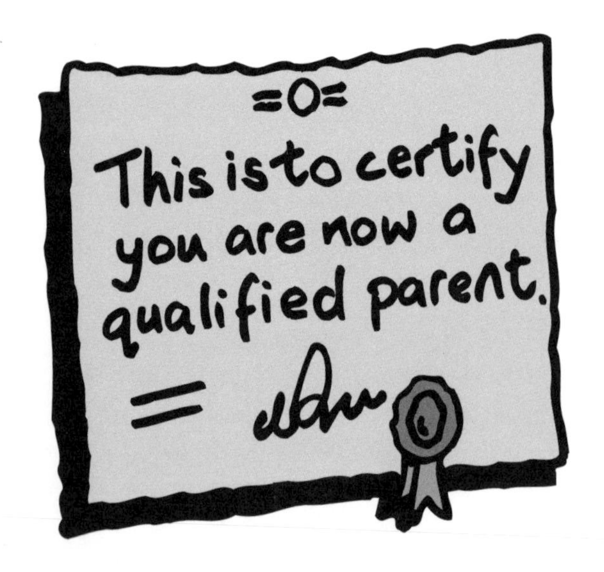

New baby shopping checklist

Basic starter pack for your baby's first few weeks

Baby clothes

- 2 packs of disposable newborn size nappies or 2 dozen terry nappies and 2 pairs of waterproof pants
- 4 to 6 vests/bodysuits
- 2 pairs socks or bootees
- 4 to 6 stretch/sleepsuits with popper legs for easy nappy access
- 10 bibs
- 2 cardigans / sweaters
- Shawl
- Hat and mittens
- 2 pairs scratch mittens
- 2 jackets or snowsuits for outdoor wear

Sleeping

- Cot and mattress – make sure the mattress fits the cot snugly
- 4 fitted cot sheets for the mattress
- 4 cot sheets
- Cot blankets (2 winter blankets – heavyweight, and 2 for summer – lightweight)

- Moses basket and/or carrycot bedding; 2 sheets, 2 fitted sheets for the mattress, 2 blankets
- Baby monitor

Remember - pillows and duvets should not be used for babies under one year old.

Breastfeeding

- 2 or 3 nursing bras
- Breast pads

Bottle feeding

- Sterilising equipment
- 250ml feeding bottles, teats and covers (6 of each)
- Infant milk formula

Baby equipment

- Changing bag with changing mat
- Baby toiletries (soap, shampoo, cotton wool, baby wipes)
- Baby bath
- Nappy bin
- Medicine chest with first-aid kit, baby paracetamol/Calpol, thermometer and nappy-rash cream
- Baby's room thermometer

Transport

- Baby buggy or pram
- Moses basket and/or carrycot
- Car seat – always buy new to ensure your baby's safety

Going into hospital

It's also a good idea to pack some items ready for when you go into hospital to have your baby. Get these ready a few weeks before the birth.

Hospital checklist for mums-to-be

- 2 or 3 front opening nightshirts/nightdresses
- Dressing gown and slippers
- 2 or 3 nursing or support bras
- 2 packs of maternity pads
- Breast pads
- 2 packs of disposable briefs
- 2 bath towels
- Toilet bag with your essential toiletries and some tissues
- An outfit for travelling home
- 4 vests/bodysuits for the baby
- Scratch mittens
- 4 stretch/sleepsuits with popper legs for easy nappy access
- Pack of nappies – for convenience use disposables for your stay in hospital
- Toiletries for your baby

We hope you enjoyed reading this book and would like to read other titles in the NSPCC range.
If you have any difficulty finding other titles you can order them direct (p&p is free) from Egmont World Limited, P O Box 7, Manchester M19 2HD.
Please make a cheque payable to Egmont World Limited and list the titles(s) you want to order on a separate piece of paper.
Please don't forget to include your address and postcode.

Thank you

… and remember every book purchased means another contribution towards the NSPCC cause.

NSPCC Child Care Guides £2.99

First-time Parent, by Faye Corlett	0 7498 4669 0
Understanding Your Baby, by Eileen Hayes	0 7498 4670 4
Understanding Your Toddler, by Eileen Hayes	0 7498 4671 2
Toddler Talk and Learning, by Ken Adams	0 7498 4776 X
Sleeping Through the Night, by Faye Corlett	0 7498 4775 1
Bullying, by Sheila Dore	0 7498 4766 2
A Special Child in the Family, by Mal Leicester	0 7498 4673 9
Being Different, by Mal Leicester	0 7498 4765 4
Potty Training and Child Development, by Faye Corlett	0 7498 4763 8
Changing Families, by Sheila Dore	0 7498 4762 X
Positive Parenting, by Eileen Hayes	0 7498 4674 7
Bedtimes and Mealtimes, by Margaret Bamforth	0 7498 4672 0

NSPCC Learning Guides £2.99
by Nicola Morgan

Get Ready for School	0 7498 4492 2
Reading and Writing at School	0 7498 4491 4

NSPCC Happy Kids Story Books £2.99
by Michaela Morgan

Maya and the New Baby.	0 7498 4637 2
Spike and the Footy Shirt	0 7498 4636 4
Jordan and the Different Day	0 7498 4638 0
Jody and the Biscuit Bully	0 7498 4635 6
Emily and the Stranger	0 7498 4639 9
Happy Kids All Together Now	0 7498 4640 2